I0410717

Survival Skills:

From Beginner to Badass. A Survival Guide with Life Saving Skills for the Wilderness or Any Dangerous Situation

Zach Williams

Table of Contents

Introduction

Congratulations on downloading *Survival Skills: From Beginner to Badass. A Survival Guide with Life Saving Skills for the Wilderness or Any Dangerous Situation* and thank you for doing so. Despite the relative comfort and safety of the modern world, mother nature is always anxious to prove just what it is she is still capable of, often at the worst possible times. Survival in these situations means being prepared with the basics every time you leave the comfort of your own home, as you never know what may happen around the next bend.

As such, the following chapters will discuss everything you need to do in order to survive should you find yourself in an unexpected survival situation, starting with utilizing a survival mindset to ensure your needs are taken care of in an appropriate order and as efficiently as possible. You will then learn all that is required to set up a proper base camp, including creating multiples types of shelter should you find yourself alone and facing the elements without a tent. With shelter out of the way, you will want to consider your options for food and water, both of which are going to be of serious concern sooner than later. With the big three covered, you will then learn various techniques for dealing with inclement weather of all sorts and natural disasters of all varieties. Finally, you will learn numerous different first aid techniques including how to make a split, use a tourniquet and perform CPR and what to do when you come into contact with poisonous plant or venomous animals.

There are plenty of books on this subject on the market, thanks again for choosing this one! Every effort was made to ensure it is full of as much useful information as possible, please enjoy!

Chapter 1: The Survival Mindset

You never know when you are going to find yourself in the middle of an emergency situation where your survival is much less assured than you are generally used to. As such, it is important to always take as many safety and survival precautions as possible, not only when you are going out into the wilderness specifically, but also if you are traveling a long distance via automobile as you never know when the worst might happen. The first thing that you are going to want to do if you find yourself in an emergency situation is to acclimate yourself to a survival mindset as quickly as possible.

A survival mindset is a mindset that is focused around ensuring that your three primary needs for survival are taken care of, to the exclusion of all else. The human body can survive for three weeks without food, three days without water and only three hours outside before dying from exposure to either extreme heat or extreme cold. With this in mind, if you find yourself in an emergency situation where help is not readily available then the first thing that you are going to want to do is to assess your situation and determine if you are in danger of succumbing to exposure. Don't be fooled by temperatures that seem somewhat temperate during the day, plan ahead and use the resources you have available to you in order to make the most of the time you have before the weather turns against you.

With shelter out of the way, it is important to consider your other needs, not just in the short term but a day, or even a week down the line depending on your situation. So much of the modern world revolves around the idea of instant gratification that you may very well find yourself sitting back and waiting for the rescue that seems certain to arrive sooner or later if you find yourself in an emergency situation. This is a strategy that is as likely to get you killed as it is to save your life, however, and convincing yourself of this fact is the first step to ensuring that you make it out of whatever it is that has befallen you alive and in one piece.

If you find yourself in a form of mild shock, then denial might seem like a perfectly reasonable response to whatever it is that has happened to you. Yes, it may be unfair or unbelievable, no, neither of those facts is going to bandage your wounds or put food in your belly until help arrives. The only way that anything is going to get done is if you stop expecting someone else to solve your problems for you and get to work making a plan for survival; afterwards, executing on that plan should be your sole mission until the situation changes.

Securing the big three

Shelter: When choosing a tent, you should always look for one that will be the most effective depending on your location. Some tents can keep you a little more insulated then others, while other tents can reflect heat from the sun making it a bit cooler inside. You also want to look for a tent that will keep out insects and water in case it rains.

Water: You also want to include a cooking set up as well as a water filtration set up. With the right equipment, you can make camping out feel almost like home.

Food: The human body can last up to three weeks without any food. During this period your body will use up any stored body fat as well as start consuming your muscle for energy. As such, in any type of survival situation, you want the number of calories that you consume to be as close to your average as possible. The average person eats between 1,500 and 2,000 calories, somewhere in that range should definitely be your goal.

During a survival situation, you are going to want to prioritize foods that are high in healthy fats. Foods containing healthy fats provide more than twice as many calories per pound when compared to foods that are primarily comprised of protein. This is why trail mix is a popular food to take on a camping trip, as the nuts are high in healthy fats and a single handful can give you several hundred calories. This is beneficial for numerous reasons, first and foremost of which is it means you don't need to bring as much with you when you are exploring out in the wilderness while also providing you with plenty of energy for all of the exercise you will be getting as well.

High calorie foods are perfect for survival because they are energy dense and your body requires a certain amount of energy per day. Any excess calories that you do consume your body will turn it into both fat and muscle, which means that if you find yourself in a situation where food is limited but you currently have too much to carry, you should try to eat as much as possible before throwing anything out. While it is perfectly natural to want and bring more traditional healthy foods with you when you are in the wilderness, the fact of the matter is that you would need to bring about five times as many vegetables and fruits as you would nuts and healthy fats to get the same result.

Here is a little food for thought, pretend that you are stranded and you can only choose between two food choices an unlimited supply of spinach, or an unlimited supply of steak. Which would you choose to eat to survive as long as possible? If you chose the spinach because you thought that it contains more nutrients then you are incorrect.

Although spinach is well known for having lots of incredible nutrients, in this case the correct answer would be the steak; an 8-ounce serving of steak might contain over 500 calories, meanwhile you would need to eat over three pounds of spinach to consume 500 calories. The spinach also lacks the amount of high quality protein that the steak provides. Your body needs that protein to rebuild muscle tissue, and heal injuries, two things that are especially important if you find yourself in a survival situation and a diet consisting of spinach will not provide those same benefits.

Also, even though spinach is a carbohydrate, your body's main source of energy, the steak, is still a better option because the protein can serve double duty by healing your body from injuries as well as powering its primary systems. By choosing animal protein you will still have the right nutrients that your body requires to survive for a good amount of time until you are either rescued or find a more abundant food source.

Chapter 2: Signaling for Help

Preparing for the worst

Before going out into a potentially dangerous area you should always contact multiple people and let them know what you are doing and when you are planning to return. It doesn't matter how competent you feel you are in an emergency scenario, just a small amount of preplanning can easily save your life. Likewise, if you plan on staying out in the wilderness for a prolonged period of time, make a schedule ahead of time and plan on checking in with the rest of the world at least once a week.

If you do find yourself in an emergency situation, the first thing that you are going to want to do is to consider how you are going to reach the outside world and let them know that you suddenly require assistance. If you are still close to civilization then there is a good chance your smart phone might still be able to get some sort of signal, solving your problems, otherwise a walkie talkie or radio might be required. Before heading on any type of multiday excursion you should always do your research and determine what level of outside communication you can expect and what radio or walkie talkie bands you can reach rescue teams on.

To ensure that when you do get in touch with rescuers, you have to be able provide them with as much information as possible; you need to keep this in mind before the moment you step into the wilderness. When you get out of your car and again when you reach your destination or make camp for the night you should mark that spot onto a map. Then, using a compass, jot down you general direction and any other coordinates you can muster. Also, note any major landmarks that you pass by, especially anything you feel will be noticeable from the air.

Finding yourself lost

If, for whatever reason, you find yourself lost then the acronym STOP can help you keep the situation from spiraling out of control.

S: Stay where you are. This is perhaps the most important thing to do if you find yourself lost in an unfamiliar place, and it is also the thing that most people fail to do. Staying in one place will always make you easier to find, as otherwise you will have no real idea if you are helping or hurting your situation. The further you walk from the point you lost your way, the less useful any of your preparations for keeping your bearings will become. The only exception to this rule is if there is an opportunity to gain an improved vantage point nearby, as this will not only help you take stock of your situation, but it will also make it easier for a rescue party to find you as well.

T: Think about everything you remember about where you have come from. You never know what details might help a rescue team find you or even help you reorient yourself so that you realize you weren't actually lost as well which is why it is important to take stock of everything you remember from the point you knew where you were to the point you found yourself lost as quickly as possible. Short term memories fade quickly, and small details, especially those you weren't paying attention to in the first place, fade more quickly still; these are the details that can literally save your life so do everything you can to solidify them in your mind ASAP.

O: Observe your surroundings. Once you have taken stock of how you ended up in your current situation the next thing that you will want to do is consider the area you currently find yourself in, specifically anything that appears as though it was made or altered by humans or any new landmarks. If you find something that is manmade then the odds of someone coming along will increase exponentially and you will have even more of a reason not to leave the area and additional landmarks will make it easier for a rescue team to find you if you do make contact with someone.

P: Plan out what you will do next. If you do find yourself in an emergency situation it is important to take the time to consider all of your various potential courses of action. The seriousness of your current situation will radically change the next steps you have to take and planning before taking further action is highly recommended.

Once you have completed the acronym you should have a relatively good idea of where you are in relation to where you went off course from your original route. If you feel as though you are extremely lost, then the best choice, as previously noted is to stay put and work on preparing the signals discussed later in this chapter. However, if you are not extremely lost and just slightly off track, then you can attempt to find your way back if you do so safely.

Above all else in this situation, your number one goal should be to ensure that you do not become any more lost than you already are. This means that the first thing you need to do is create a starting point, it can be a nearby rock formation, spray paint, a piece of clothing hung on a branch or whatever you will remember as your starting point. After that you should leave a trail behind you as you go. A trail can be made up of bits of cloth hung from trees, bent branches or even by dragging a stick on a ground if the location permits. If you realize that your first attempt has failed, then just simply follow your trail back to your starting point and move in a different direction. Before you set out in a given direction it is important to have a clear idea in mind of what it is you are backtracking to, only by having a specific idea when it comes to success or failure will you ever end up helping your cause instead of hurting it.

Rescue signals

When extremely lost and staying put, you are going to want to consider how to meet all of your basic survival needs first and foremost, including the creation of a temporary shelter as there is no telling how long you are going to have to fend for yourself until help arrives. First things first, however, you are going to want to create a signal that shows any other humans in the area that something is amiss.

Visual Signals: Assuming you have the required tools, there is nothing better than a signal fire for indicating that humans are present. The ideal signal fire is one that can produce thick black smoke which makes it very easy to spot even from a distance. To create a signal fire, you need to start with a large regular fire, but it is important to not become too overzealous and create a fire that you cannot control. This fire should be in plain view, in an elevated spot if possible, so that rescuers can spot the light and smoke from the greatest distance allowable.

Once this fire is started you want to then add in something that will cause the smoke to turn as thick and black as possible. The best choices for this are going to be either motor oil, brake fluid, or plastic. If none of these are available then you can also cover the fire with freshly cut tree branches with the leaves still on it, the greener the better. If you ever have to leave the signal fire while it is burning, even for a little while, it is important to leave a note or some indication that you are still in the area to prevent you from accidentally missing your rescuers.

While not as useful as a full blown signal fire, a mirror is a compact and useful way to get the attention of someone in the distance assuming there is enough light to generate a reflection. A small mirror takes up practically nothing in your daily carry which makes it a must have whenever you are venturing into the wilderness. If a mirror is unavailable you can also use tin foil, aluminum cans, and other shiny objects that reflect light. At night time a flashlight or laser pointer can also be effective.

Audio signals: Screaming and yelling will not be very effective if help is not an earshot away, so including an emergency whistle in your camping gear can save the strain on your voice and get the attention of someone further away as well. Gun shots are also very effective in getting the attention of others. With all these signals, there is a rule of three that should be followed for the best results. This means that you are going to want to create noise in bursts of three that are spaced five seconds apart. This will signal others in the area that you are in distress and also provide them the time they need to create a response noise that is not drowned out by your own noise.

Chapter 3: Creating a Base Camp

Setting up a base camp is almost mandatory in most survival situations as it allows for ease of access to all of your available equipment and also provides protection from the elements if required.

Basics

Choosing a location: When setting up a camp site you need to have it in a safe location away from any predators and also not in the path of any streams that might form should it happen to rain which means being on the lookout for the signs you might be in a riverbed, even a fallow one. If you are expecting rescue in the form of an airplane, then you may want to set up somewhere in the open so you can be spotted easily. However, if you do so you will then need to be extra wary of thunderstorms and at the first sign of them take your tent down and move to a location where you are not the tallest point in the area. Ideally you will want to choose a location that has clear sightlines in as many directions as possible.

Setting up camp: If you find yourself out in the wild without a tent then a the very least you are going to want to find a way to raise yourself off the ground as much as possible at night. Not only will this dramatically increase the amount of warmth that you will be able to retain (the ground will get extremely cold in most places), it will also help protect you from all manner of crawling creatures that bite and may carry diseases. If you have food with you then it is important to always store it away from the rest of your camp and out of the reach of animals; since you never know how long you will have to stretch the food that you do have, it's best to avoid sharing if possible. Remember, many animals are naturally wary of unfamiliar smells which means that if you urinate around the perimeter of your camp you will have fewer unwanted visitors. Finally, when it comes to taking care of bodily functions it is important to choose a spot to defecate that is at least 50 feet downwind from your camp and to always bury your leavings to avoid attracting animals.

Additionally, there are numerous different types of shelters that you can create depending on what materials you are lucky enough to have hanging around. First and foremost, if you have a tarp or other large, heavy piece of material then you can easily make a perfectly serviceable tend with just a piece of rope and a few rocks. If you don't have a rope, a thick branch will also work. All you need to do is find a pair of trees that are the appropriate distance apart, position the rope or branch between them and then drape the material over the branch. A few rocks to secure the bottom edge will leave you with a passable shelter that will protect you from the sun and rain and provide a little extra insulation against the cold as well.

When it comes to placing the rope or branch into the neighboring trees, it is important to place it relatively close to the ground so that you can do little more than sleep in the space. The less space that the tent covers, the easier it will be to warm up using just your body heat. If you are using this method to protect yourself from snow, it is important to try and create a steeper roof to your tent to encourage the snow to roll off of it more easily.

If you aren't lucky enough to have a tarp or tarp-equivalent with you then you are going to instead want to construct a simple lean-to in order to shelter yourself from the elements. To start, you are going to want to look for something long and big enough, think boulder or fallen tree, which you are then going to lean other things up against in a horizontal fashion. With a base to build from established, the next thing that you will want to do is find a number of large branches to lean against the base to create support for the smaller items you will eventually use for insulation. Just like with the tent, the lower you can keep the lean-to to the ground, the better. Finally, you will want to insulate your lean-to using fallen leaves, grasses, moss, anything that you can fill in the space between the branches with, the more the merrier. Anything added in this stage will improve the level of insulation your lean-to would provide.

Depending on the conditions that you find yourself in, you may also want to position your fire pit underneath your lean-to for additional warmth. This is only recommended in areas that are somewhat damp, however, as your lean-to will otherwise quite likely be a fire hazard. If you are planning to put your fire pit into the lean-to it is important to construct the space with this in mind and not decide to add it in after the fact. The fire should be positioned near the opening to your lean-to in order to provide it with the proper amount of ventilation to prevent you from constantly inhaling smoke.

Creating a fire: The ability to start a fire is one of the most valuable skills that you can possess in any survival situation. The easiest way to ensure that you are always prepared to start a fire is to ensure that you have a flint and steel as well as a few cotton balls that have been soaked in petroleum jelly. The cotton ball trick is extremely useful because they are very light and there is no excuse not to carry them with you and they will start a fire in windy conditions and even in the middle of a rainstorm.

To light the cotton balls, you want to strike the flint in a downwards motion onto the flint with the steel, this strike will result in sparks which should ideally contact your flammable material. You will want to have additional kindling in the form of dry grass, or ideally a bird's nest so that once the cotton balls light you can keep the fire going. Once your flammable material is lit and you start to see embers and a little bit of smoke forming this is when you need to protect it from the wind using your body and hands and blow on it gently enough to start the fire. As the fire gets bigger, you will need to add firewood and other things that you will use to keep the fire going. Carrying a carbon fiber knife that has a flint in the case will allow you to not only start fires but also be prepared for a wide variety of additional emergencies.

Creating a space for cooking: A cooking setup can be used for many purposes like boiling water, and cooking food as well as keeping your fire contained and productive. To make a cooking setup you need to start with a traditional fire pit. From there, you will want to track down three thick tree branches that are not so dry that they will catch on fire from the heat. Branches that are roughly half your height tend to work most effectively.

With the branches already picked out you will want to then dig three holes in a triangular shape around your fire pit that are large enough to hold the branches put small enough to hold them tightly. Once they are in place you will want to angle them towards the center of the fire pit and fill in the excess space with dirt so it supports the weight of the branch. Ideally you will want the three branches to overlap with one another at the top while leaving enough space for the pot or other cooking apparatus you plan to use. Once you have this all set up you can hang a pot above these sticks and cook or boil whatever you need.

You should avoid using plastic as a base to cook with because it will melt and it will cause black smoke to form which is unhealthy to inhale and ingest. If you don't have a cooking pot available, then shaping tin foil (which is highly recommended to always carry with you) into it a pot is known to work in a pinch.

Chapter 4: Finding Food and Water

Food

Basics: Anything with fur and feathers is safe to eat as long as it is cooked thoroughly. The only exception to this is carrion dwellers and other scavengers as they are prone to carrying a host of diseases that make them more trouble than they are worth. To ensure that the meat is cooked thoroughly you want to cut into the raw meat and take note of its color before cooking. Meat that is safe to go ahead and cook should be either white, pink, or red. You will know it is finished cooking when you no longer see that color anywhere inside of it.

Cooking the meat will make it much safer than normal, though this is still not a complete guarantee depending on the state of the animal prior to its consumption. It is important to take the time to observe the animal you are planning to kill in its natural state when possible to ensure that it is exhibiting normal behavior. Animals experiencing aberrant behavior should be avoided as this can be a sign of serious illness. While you can realistically consume nearly the entirety of any animal that you kill, if you are not practiced at the act you will find sticking to the primary cuts of meat easier to handle. Additionally, you will only want to store cooked meat for 24-28 hours to ensure it remains a healthy choice as well.

Seafood: If you find yourself near a lake or the ocean, then are practically guaranteed a reliable source of protein if you approach the task smartly. Remember, it is very dangerous to eat fish that live in polluted water so if there is any doubt in your mind it is better to be safe than sorry. Additionally, it is important to always cook the fish before eating it to kill any bacteria or parasites it might be home to. In fact, it is illegal in the U.S. to serve raw fish that has not been previously frozen. If relying on fish from the saltwater avoid eating fish that live in the reefs and close to shore as most of them contain ciguatera which is dangerous to humans. Even larger fish that feed off of reef fish will contain ciguatera, a form of food poisoning.

If you are far out at sea, then most fish caught out there is safe to eat raw. However, avoid cowfish, oil fish, red snapper, jack, porcupine fish, trigger fish, puffer fish, and thorn fish because these species tend to have poisonous flesh.

Crustaceans such as shrimp and crayfish are safe to eat as long as they are cooked thoroughly. Mollusks such as octopus and shellfish are also safe. Just note that mussels in tropical areas during summer could be dangerous to consume, as well as any shellfish that stays above water during a high tide.

Looking outside the normal spectrum: If more traditional supplies of meat are unavailable in the area you find yourself in, this does not mean you can lay off of the protein, especially in a strenuous situation. This means you may need to resort to eating insects and other small animals you might not consider traditional food sources. Many insects can be dangerous so you should avoid eating spiders, caterpillars, brightly colored insects, flies, mosquitos, ticks, and adult insects that sting and bite. Worms are safe to eat, just place them in a container of clean water and they will wash themselves out. Remember, insects that have hard shells on the outside must be cooked first before consuming, others can be consumed raw.

Amphibians such as frogs and salamanders are safe options as well, however, it is important that you do not confuse toads for frogs as toads are poisonous. You can tell a frog from a toad because they are going to be more brightly colored and many poisonous varieties have a pattern that looks like an X on its back. Additionally, you will be able to tell a frog by its long, relatively thin legs and body while a toad's legs are going to be much more short and stout. Additionally you will always be able to tell a frog is a frog if you see it leap from place to place as toads prefer to crawl. If you have caught an amphibian and aren't sure which is which you can look at the feet, if they are webbed then what you have caught is likely safe to eat. You can find frogs and amphibians near ponds and bodies of water.

If you are out in the wild, plants can be a good food source if you don't have other options. However, much like amphibians, many plants are extremely toxic for humans which means that when in doubt you are going to want to avoid plants you are unsure of. If you absolutely must try out unknown berries, then there is a three-step process you can follow to do so relatively safely. This process is by no means safe in a conventional sense and should only be attempted when you literally have no other options. Additionally, you will want to pick out a plant that you can easily find a lot of it as it's not worth it to test a plant that won't even fill you up once.

Once you find a plant that you are curious to learn if it is edible, the first step is to rub it onto your skin. If nothing happens, you will then want to wait at least five minutes and mash plant until it starts to produce a liquid, and then rub that onto your skin as well. If this also yields no negative results then the next thing you will want to do is press it to your lips, wait, put it in your mouth, wait and then finally chew up the plant but make sure not to swallow it. If you still do not feel that anything is wrong, then you can swallow only a tiny amount of the plant and then let it digest completely for about 12 hours. After that try eating a larger amount and waiting again before tentatively considering the experiment a success.

When trying this method out it is very important if at any time of the testing you feel a burning sensation, or feel ill after swallowing, to immediately discontinue the testing and induce vomiting if possible. Before attempting this test, you should allow your body to go eight hours without eating first to ensure the most accurate results. If possible, you should also attempt to cook the plants beforehand as some plants, but not all, lose their toxicity when cooked.

Berries can either be very poisonous or cause no harm at all. Unless you are an expert you should only stick to eating blackberries and raspberries. There are too many poisonous berries to go into detail on so never eat a berry that you are uncertain of. If you are in an urgent situation where you are starving and berries are the only thing available you should still abstain from eating them.

Mushrooms, just like berries can be very poisonous or completely benign. As such, if you have any questions about the mushrooms you are considering consuming it is much better to take precautions than suffer the effects of poisoning or even death. When looking for mushrooms look at the bottom of the cap, also called the skirt, and see if it is either white or is producing a liquid when touched. If the bottom is white or lactates, then you should avoid the mushroom at all costs. Red mushrooms are also very dangerous and should never be consumed.

If you decide to eat a mushroom, unless you are completely certain it is safe, cook it first and then take it through the three step process for testing potentially poisonous plants. Even a small amount of a poisonous mushroom can be very damaging to your body if ingested so use extreme caution when testing.

Water

The most important thing you need to survive for a prolonged period of time in the wilderness is water. It doesn't matter where you are going, if there is a possibility that you might be staying long than intended, do yourself a favor and bring as much water with you as you possibly can. Even with these precautions, however, if you find yourself in an emergency situation they are likely not going to be enough which is where the tips outlined in the remainder of this chapter come in.

Water follows the path of least resistance in a downward slope which means that if you are searching for water you are going to want to seek out the lowest point you possibly can. If you find yourself in a pond that has dried up, by digging into the soil you may find water hidden below the surface. If you can find mud, then you will know that water is nearby. Once you do find water, however, it is important to never drink from it directly unless you literally have no other choice, and even then, only if the water is flowing. In all scenarios, you are going to be better off holding out to purify the water if that is even a remote possibility.

Water purification: The simplest way to purify water is to create a basic filter. This can be done by taking a wet piece of cloth and then covering it with a layer of charcoal, a layer of cleaned gravel and a layer of fresh grass. With this setup, you get four layers of filtering that will clean water that was already somewhat healthy. The grass will remove the big things in the water while the gravel, charcoal, and cloth removes the much smaller things. You simply hold this filter over a container that you wish to store your filtered water in then just pour water slowly through the filter.

Whenever possible you are then going to want to take the water that has been filtered in this way and then boil it for a minimum of 60 seconds. If bacteria in the water is killed after a minute of boiling water, then additional heat isn't going to affect it. After you have boiled the water, the next thing you will ideally want to do is to chemically purify it as well. If you have them, a very small amount of bleach or iodine are great for this and all you will need to add is about four drops of these chemicals per quart of cold or murky water, and if you have warm or clear water then you will just need two drops. Give the water a shake and let it sit for about half an hour. If you want to be extra safe you could put that water into a clear plastic water bottle and let it sit in the sun for a few hours as this will cause it to vaporize and then condense again leaving the remaining water as pure as possible.

If you are preparing for an excursion into the wilderness, then a steripen may be a useful investment. The steripen emits an ultraviolet light that kills bacteria when flashed into the water, rendering virtually any water drinkable with no muss or fuss. You may find it overwhelming, but it is important to take all the steps that you can to ensure that the water is as clean as possible before drinking because a common symptom for most waterborne diseases is diarrhea. Diarrhea is a sure way to get dehydrated fast, and if you try to make up for your dehydrated state by drinking even more contaminated water then you could be headed towards a life threatening situation.

The three primary waterborne illnesses to look out for include giardia, cryptosporidium, and E. coli. Giardia and cryptosporidium are both parasites unlike E. coli, which is a bacteria. Symptoms of these conditions are abdominal cramps, watery stools, bloating, lack of appetite, fever, and vomiting. These conditions are also hard to detect early on because you do not start to get symptoms until a few days after ingesting contaminated water.

Aside from looking for ponds, lakes, rivers, and streams there are also other methods of obtaining water, although they are slower and more complicated as well. Tree tapping is a good way to get ready to drink water, though it should be consumed in moderation as it will contain sugar that makes it difficult for your body to perform other important functions optimally. To get water from a tree you have to get a knife and dig out a small hole. You should try to make the hole as small as possible and still be able to get water out because by doing this method you are causing permanent damage to that tree. Once you cut a hole into the tree you should notice that it is leaking water. If it is, then just dig a little bit more and move on to the second step.

For this step, you need to get a small piece of wood and shape it to the size of a pencil. Then you want to sharpen both sides of this pencil shaped wood with a knife. Once that is done by using a rock, something hard, or brute force jam this piece of wood into the hole at an angle so that water can drip down from it. If water is dripping down, then you know that you have done this correctly. From this point, you can just hold your water bottle there or tie it to the tree in place. This is a long process and will take hours before it fills up a canteen. Although this method will only work on some trees like maple, sycamore, and birch trees.

Fern plants are also good sources of water. Find a fern plant and dig around its roots you should eventually find what looks like a tiny potato growing on the roots. This should be about the size of gumball and should contain a decent amount of water for its size.

Solar stills are also a good way to get water with very little resources and a lot of time. All you need for this is the sun, a container to store water in, a plastic bag, and some fresh leaves. Start off by digging a hole into the ground, it has to be about arm's length deep, and wide enough to fit two basketballs. Next, you will need to find some fresh leaves and crush them up slightly before placing them at the bottom of hole. Be careful to only use leaves from a plant that you have already confirmed not to be poisonous. Next, place your container on top of those leaves, this container should be small so that it only covers about half of the total space.

You will then want to cover the hole with plastic, held in place by a number of heavy rocks. With the plastic secure, you will then want to place another rock in the center that is heavy enough to weigh down the plastic towards the container. The way this works is that the sun will cause the moisture in the leaves to rise, and since there is a plastic bag over the leaves, it will get trapped onto the plastic bag; if the plastic bag is angled correctly, it will let the water slide into your container so you can have fresh drinking water.

Another way to do this same method is to find a bush or a tree branch full of leaves and stick as much of that branch into the plastic bag as possible and tie a knot at the beginning of the bag. Make sure that this solar still is in direct contact with the sun and that the leaves of the plant you are using are not toxic.

The last method you can use to get water is by cutting out the sleeves of a shirt and tying them to your ankles. Once you do this, you simply walk over a field of grass and the fabric of the shirt sleeves should collect water. After you collect enough water you can take the sleeves off your ankle and suck the moisture out of them. While this won't be enough to keep you completely hydrated it will be enough to keep you going while you work on a more permanent solution.

Chapter 5: Dealing with the Elements

The human body can only withstand a prolonged internal body temperature of close to 37 degrees Celsius or 98.6 Fahrenheit. Even if your internal body temperature drops by just a few degrees you will start to become hypothermic and when it rises over by a few degrees you become hyperthermic.

Hypothermia is a result of your internal body temperature dropping too low. As hypothermia gets worse, your heart, nervous system, and other bodily functions will stop working properly. Hypothermia can eventually lead to death if left untreated. Symptoms include shivering, lack of coordination, faster breathing, and a faster heartrate. As hypothermia gets worse you will experience extreme shivering, progressive loss of consciousness, slow/shallow breathing, and a weak pulse.

If you are afraid you are in the early stages of hypothermia, the first thing that you will need to do is to remove any wet clothes and do everything you can to get warm. If fresh clothing and blankets are not available, then you are going to at least want to keep moving to keep your circulation up.

Hyperthermia is a result of your internal body temperature rising too far above normal. As your temperature rises even further you will experience heat waves, followed by heat exhaustion which results in heavy sweating and a rapid pulse, then eventually heat stroke which is the most severe and dangerous. If left untreated it causes damage to the brain and other important organs and can eventually lead to death. To prevent hyperthermia from taking place you must limit your body's exposure to high temperatures as much as possible. It is also important to stay well hydrated. To avoid becoming overheated during your exposure it is important to limit physical activity to the periods of early morning or late afternoon and always cover as much of your skin as possible when in direct sunlight. Pace yourself and take things slowly and you should be fine.

Ways to regulate body temperature: It is impossible to control the weather but it is possible to control your response to it. If you plan on going into the cold, then always wear a thick layer of clothing. If possible, make the outermost layer waterproof because if your clothes are wet then they will get cold faster. Always have a source of wood around you so that you can start a fire at moment's notice.

If you plan on going into a hot environment, then always wear enough clothing so that the majority of your skin is protected from the sun, but take care to wear light fabrics lest you overheat. If you are stranded and waiting for help, then try as much as possible to find shade and to not move around. By moving around, your body is burning calories which also raises your body heat.

Rainstorm: A rainstorm is not much of a threat compared to other storms but it does pose some unique problems nevertheless. First and foremost, it is important to get a lay of the land to ensure you are not at risk for a flash flood should the storm continue apace. A rain storm also sets you up for hypothermia if you are caught unaware.

If you are out camping, then taking cover under a tree or in your tent would be your best bet. If there are any holes in your tent, you can easily patch it up with duct tape. If you are out hiking, then the safest option is to either cancel the hike or wait until the rainstorm ends. Although it all depends on the hike, if it is on a trail then that is not much of a problem. However, if there is rock climbing involved then the rocks could still be slippery even hours after the rain stops.

If you find yourself in a thunderstorm, then the best place to be is either in amongst a large group of trees or in a vehicle if you are going to be the tallest object around otherwise. While this might seem counterintuitive, the rubber tires on the vehicle will ground it making lightning strikes irrelevant. In case of a flash flood you still want to follow the same rules as thunderstorms, but at the same time you need to avoid being on low ground, especially around streams and valleys. It doesn't take much water to sweep you or your gear away so avoid crossing any streams with strong currents as much as possible, however if you must then make sure that the stream does not go higher than your knees.

If you are driving during a flash flood, then never drive into a body of water unless you know how deep it is. If you drive into water that is too deep, you risk floating the car. Once that happens, you have no control over your vehicle, and if that body of water leads off a cliff then that is where your car is going.

If there is hail, then the size of the hail will determine what needs to be done. In some cases, hail can form to as big as golf balls and travel at speeds over 100 miles per hour. That is equivalent to a baseball player throwing a golf ball at your head. But chances of that are rare, so if a hailstorm does occur, pick up a piece of hail on the ground, and proceed to determine if you should ignore it or find a shelter.

Sand: If you are caught in a sandstorm, then the best thing to do is to seek shelter immediately. If you have a tent that is strong enough, then that should be just fine. However, if you are nowhere near shelter, then you must cover all openings found on your head (mouth, ears and nose to a certain extent) as well as your eyes. If you have goggles and a mask that filters out small particles, then that should work. However, it is not wise to continue your path if a sandstorm is occurring because you could get lost from your original trail and things will be flying around inside the sandstorm that could injure you. Waiting until a sandstorm passes is the smartest choice.

Quicksand has a wet cement like consistency and when stepped in it is extremely difficult to get out of. The more you struggle the deeper it pulls you in. Most of the times however, people don't die a result of suffocating but because of the extreme heat of the sun shining on them for hours and hours. To get out of quicksand or to help someone out of it, you should never offer them your hand because there is a chance that they can pull you in or dislocate a shoulder. If available, use a stick or if alone try to reach for anything that you can grab onto that you can use to pull yourself out with. Make your way to the edges of the quicksand and try to get one leg out of it and once that is done try monkey crawling along the hard sand until you break free

Once out, however, you should not walk because there will still be a lot of sand, rocks, and other debris inside your clothes and if you tried to, you will quickly get extreme rashes or boils from all the rubbing and friction. When you get out, take off your clothes and shoes and shake out and remove as much stuff from the inside of your items to avoid getting rashes. After removing as many particles as possible, quickly put your clothes back on to protect yourself from the sun.

Water: Learning how to swim should be mandatory if you plan to go anywhere near water but some people don't think that drowning will happen to them. If you encounter someone drowning, unless you are a trained lifeguard you should not attempt to swim after them because in a panic the drowning victim could try to use you for flotation and end up drowning you instead. Always look for a rope or a stick to drag them into shore instead as this is much more effective. Only if the person is unconscious should you go into the water to save them because they no longer pose a threat of drowning you. What you want to do is swim to them and drag them closer and closer to shore. When you get them to shore and they are unresponsive then you want to immediately perform CPR.

Chapter 6: Surviving a Natural Disaster

Natural disasters can be life threatening both during the event and for several days afterwards. Aside from preparing for them beforehand, there are things that you must do in the midst of the crisis and afterwards to ensure the survival of yourself and the others around you.

Earthquakes: Earthquakes are caused when underground faults are broken and the pressure buildup is released in the form of seismic waves which cause the ground to shake. Buildings and houses are very dangerous places to be in during an earthquake. At the first sign of an earthquake, the safest place to be is out in the open with no structures around you; this is because during an earthquake the building or house could collapse while you are still inside of it and can lead to serious injury or death.

If you find yourself trapped in a building or house while an earthquake is happening and the exit is blocked or too far away, then the first step you should take is to take cover under something sturdy. Your best bet is to either look for the closest bathroom, doorframe, or anything else that is likely to offer protection in the event of damage to the foundation of the building.

Once the earthquake has stopped it is still dangerous to be in the building or house, because it may have loosened up the foundation and the entire thing could collapse at any moment. The first thing you need to do is help secure everyone out of the building or home as fast as possible and to leave unimportant things behind because you can always go back for them later. After everyone is safe outside you need to wait there for a couple hours because another earthquake could occur and the secondary round of damage is likely to be much more intense than the first.

Hurricanes: Hurricanes are caused when rising warm moist air displaces cold air high above the atmosphere. Hurricanes are extremely dangerous and luckily today we have the technology to track them and find out where they are likely to occur. By keeping up to date with the news and paying attention to warnings in the weather you should be able to prepare for one early enough to protect you, your family, and your belongings. Strong buildings and basements are excellent places to hide while a hurricane is passing by as they offer a lot of protection.

Weak houses and buildings should be evacuated weeks or days prior to the arrival of the hurricane, because hurricanes can have wind speeds of over 100 miles per hour which can easily rip a ceiling right off of an old home. If you are unprepared and a hurricane does arrive, never go outside unless you are moving to a safer location. Standing outside is very dangerous because during a hurricane, debris is flying around everywhere and you can easily be hit with something that can cause serious injury. Even if you don't believe your home will hold up to a hurricane it is still better to be inside of it then outside however while inside of it you need to find a spot that you believe offers the most protection. Find anything strong and sturdy that you can take cover under that can withstand parts of the ceiling falling on top of. It should also be really heavy or attached to the floor so that the hurricane does not pick it up.

During a hurricane, many stores, hotels, apartment complexes, schools, and other buildings will allow people to take shelter until the hurricane passes by. These places offer free food and water and will also broadcast the news so that you know when it is safe to return to your homes.

Floods and Tsunamis: The result of multiple powerful waves crashing onto the shore of a beach, tsunamis will destroy and carry almost everything in its path. Inside of a tsunami will be a lot of very harmful debris that the tsunami picked up from houses, trees, cars, and other things that are on the ground.

Shorelines and the areas next to beaches are extremely dangerous places to be during a tsunami as they are most vulnerable to destruction. The best possible way of ensuring safety is to get to higher ground. Buildings and houses have a risk of being destroyed however some houses if they are strong enough will stay put but the inside of the house will be flooded. The worst case scenario would be if a tsunami is arriving and you do not have enough time to move to higher ground; if such event happens, then you want to get a ladder and have everybody climb up to the roof of the house and stay put.

Avalanche: When snow on a mountain that was perfectly balanced becomes disturbed, thousands of pounds of compact snow comes rushing down the mountain. An avalanche can be extremely scary because you will usually see and hear it coming but will not have enough time to run away from it. If you ever plan on going out in the snow always go with friends and always bring a GPS tracking device with you. After an avalanche, it is likely that you will be trapped under compact snow and not have much room to move or breathe, which can eventually lead to death from suffocation as the snow takes the consistency of almost cement.

To maximize your chance of survival you want to always be strapped with someone else so either they can find you or you can find them, and before the avalanche does hit you want to make a pocket of air by covering your head. Then take a deep breath of air and brace for impact. If possible, try grabbing onto a nearby tree or boulder. During the passing of the avalanche, if you happen to be swept away try your best to swim upwards to stay as close to the top of the snow as possible. Before you get buried, stick one hand in the air so that you can have a sense of direction where the surface is.

People stuck in snow might be disoriented and not know which way they should be digging so you can try spitting and see which way gravity pulls your saliva. Also, try your best to dig out a breathing area in front of your face, this should supply you with at least 30 minutes for rescuers to come and get you. If you know that you are buried deep, then try your best to conserve your breath because it is almost impossible to dig through the snow with your bare hands. If you happen to have a snow shovel, then you can give that a try as well. Being patient and waiting for help is the only thing you can do in some situations.

Tornado: Tornadoes almost never appear without a warning and are classified either from F-0 to F-5. F-0 being only a mild tornado and F-5 being the most destructive. Tornadoes can get powerful enough to lift up cars and wipe out houses so they should always be taken seriously and preparation should always be done before a tornado is expected to arrive.

You should always stay clear of the path of a tornado as much as possible, and you definitively have to take immediate action and drive to a safer location ahead of time. If at home and a tornado is likely coming your way, then you need to find a safe spot in your house. Look for areas in the center of the house and in small rooms. Also, stay away from the outsides walls of the house and from windows because there is a chance that the tornado can throw debris right through them. Basements are also safe places to take shelter in case of a tornado because the entire house is a shield for that one area.

When outside during a tornado try to get as low to the ground as possible and if you can, then get inside of a ditch and take cover there. If inside of a vehicle, always get out of it because a tornado can easily tip it over or pick it up and throw it in another direction. However, if you are far enough away from the tornado you should also attempt to drive away from its path; if you are on a road that allows you to go over 60 miles per hour, you can most likely outrun the tornado.

Chapter 7: First Aid Techniques

When you find yourself facing an emergency that is going to require first aid, the first thing you will want to remember is that remaining calm in any situation, no matter how severe, is the most important thing to do. By remaining calm you are preventing yourself from doing anything foolish that will worsen the situation. You also have the time to think out the best course of action you need to take. If you ever find yourself in a emergency just understand that the problem is only as bad as you think it is and you are not the only one to have ever been in that situation.

Cuts and broken bones: Cuts, bites, and scratches from wild animals should always be cleaned out with clean water first or preferably a disinfectant, then you want to stop the bleeding with whatever you have available at the time (strips of cloth work great for this purpose). Every few hours you should change the bandages. Fractures and broken bones can be a little more serious, as the victim is usually unable to move on their own. To treat a fracture until help arrives you need to move the injured to a safe location and stop any bleeding by creating a tourniquet followed by a splint

If you are dealing with a person who is bleeding excessively, then ideally you are going to want to use sterile gauze to apply pressure directly to the wound. Only when this is unavailable do you want to use what is known as homemade dressing, aka anything that is not gauze, since you can actually make the situation worse by adding elements that can lead to infection into the wound. Still, if you are in the middle of nowhere a shirt that might not be the cleanest is certainly better than bleeding to death. If a steady supply of pressure is not enough to stop the bleeding completely, the next thing that you will want to do is use a tourniquet.

Create a tourniquet: While the use of a tourniquet has critics on both sides of the issue, the truth of the matter is that as long as the tourniquet is applied properly and not left on unnecessarily, then it can easily save a person's life with little to no negative side effects. While concerns of nerve damage and limb loss are not unfounded, recent studies show that less than half of one percent of all people who are treated for blood loss via the use of a tourniquet require limb amputation because of the tourniquet and less than two percent of all people experience any type of nerve damage. Damage from prolonged tourniquet use doesn't begin for upwards of two hours, and upwards of eight hours of continuous use are required before amputation becomes a realistic option.

While a professionally made tourniquet is nice to have, it is hardly a practical addition to your daily carry, especially as there are so many other things can be used for the same purpose in a pinch. The belt at your waist, a long sleeve shirt, shoe laces, bicycle tubing, the strap from your backpack or even a bra are all ready-made for tourniquet duty should the need arise. Along with an object to act as a makeshift tourniquet, you are also going to need something to keep it tight, officially known as a torsion device. What you are looking for here is anything that is long and thin; if you are in the wilderness then there are likely to be plenty of sticks in the area that will work just fine.

When it comes to applying a tourniquet, it is important to only use it on limbs and never the neck; this may seem self-explanatory, but people tend not to think clearly during a crisis. For starters, you are going to want to wrap the tourniquet around the affected limb about two inches towards your core from where the wound occurred, taking special care to avoid joints or major arteries. When in doubt, move closer to your core as opposed to further away.

With the positioning completed you will then want to tie the tourniquet in place using a single knot tied overhand; you will then want to set the torsion device directly on top of the knot before tying it in place with either a square know or another knot tied overhand.

Create a splint: If you find that you need to create a splint to deal with an injured party member, the first thing that you will need to do is find something that is rigid enough to ensure the fractured area remains stabilized. Something made of wood is the most common approach, though even a rolled newspaper will work in a pinch. When it comes to securing the splint to the afflicted area you are going to want to consult the list of items that can be uses as a tourniquet because they can all pull double duty as splint fasteners as well.

Don't forget to attend to any bleeding prior to dealing with anything in need of a split. Likewise, never move an injured individual without applying a splint as this will almost always cause the injury to become more severe. With that in mind, you are going to want to set the split so that it reaches far enough above the afflicted area to align with the nearest joint on either side. As such, if you needed to splint your forearm, you would want the splint to reach from your wrist to your elbow. When you tie the splint on, you will want to ensure that it is tight enough to prevent undue movement and loose enough to prevent a loss of blood flow. Finally, once the splint has been properly secured it is important to check it regularly to ensure that it is not cutting off blood flow, as the area might already be numb and a change might not be noticed otherwise.

If you need to put one of your hand, or someone else's, into a splint then the first thing that you will want to do is to ball up something soft and place it in the palm of the hand that has been injured to give it a bit of structure for the remainder of the split. Once the fingers of the hand are closed around the object, the next thing you are going to want to do is wrap the entirety of the hand in a large cloth, leaving just the finger tips exposed. This cloth should move in a horizontal direction across the hand starting at the thumb and moving towards the pinky. With this done, you will then want to ensure the hand is bound properly using additional ties, taking care to not make things so tight that they cut off circulation.

Burns: To treat a burn, you have to identify the cause of the burn and act accordingly. Burns from the cold temperature should be warmed by placing the area of the burn in warm water or by blowing warm air on the burn. Burns from hot liquid should be cooled by running cold water over it for 10-

20 minutes and never use ice. If someone is burned from being electrocuted, then you should separate them from the current and immediately check for a pulse and apply CPR if necessary. With the torsion device in place, you will then want to rotate it so the tourniquet tightens against the limb just until the point where bleeding stops, it is important to not put more constraints on the limb than necessary, so stop the moment the blood loss subsides. Finally, you will want to ensure the torsion device is going to remain in place by taking the ends of the second knot and tying it to the limb and the tourniquet respectively.

Choking: Choking is a fatal accident that can happen anytime you are eating. First aid for choking starts off with giving five back thrusts which is basically using the palm of your hand and hitting in between the person's shoulder blades. After that is done you want to perform five abdominal thrusts (also known as the Heimlich maneuver). To do the Heimlich maneuver you need to stand behind the person and give them a bear hug with your hands on their belly button and pull in an upwards angle. This process should be repeated until the person can breathe regularly.

CPR: Cardiopulmonary Resuscitation should be performed immediately if someone has little nor no pulse and is unresponsive. This could be a result of drowning, electrocution, poisoning, or fainting. The first step is to call for medical help immediately and then begin CPR. By performing CPR you are allowing oxygenated blood to flow around the body of the victim. Without this oxygenated blood, the brain is not receiving any oxygen and in only a matter of minutes the victim's brain will start to receive serious damage. It only takes eight minutes without blood flow for the brain to die.

After help is on the way to you, the next thing to do is to position the person in need of CPR on their back with their head facing the sky and tilt their head at an angle to ensure that their airway is unrestricted. You will then want to put your hands on their sternum and, with your arms straight, push onto the person's sternum 30 times in a quick manner. This step is called the chest compressions and the amount of strength used should vary depending on who is receiving CPR chest compressions should be administered at a rate of 100 pumps per minute. For young children and old people, you should use little force as their ribs may break. When performing chest compressions your patient's ribs may break during the process, so as soon as you start hearing the cracking you want to immediately stop the compressions for a few seconds and then resume the process.

After performing 30 chest compressions, the next step is to breathe for the person. First, you want to make sure that their chin is up and head tilted back to clear all airways into the victim's lungs. Next, pinch the nostrils and make an airtight seal with your lips onto your patient's and breathe into them. You should also keep an eye over the chest of the victim and see if it is rising up and down as you breathe into them. You need to apply two breaths and immediately start doing chest compressions again. This should be repeated over and over until help arrives or the victim starts responding and is breathing on their own.

Poison and venom: If you feel that you or someone else has ingested or otherwise come into contact with a poisonous plant, then immediate action is required as time is of the essence. The first thing to do is to recognize the symptoms. Someone who is poisoned may be confused or behave in an erratic fashion, they may have difficulty breathing, exhibit signs of vomiting, or have a redness or overall discoloration around their face and hands. If you are not in a position to get traditional medical attention, the first thing that you will want to do is to induce vomiting. After that, you need to rinse out the mouth of the victim with water. If poisoned on the skin, then you need to get soap and water and rinse it out for 15 – 20 minutes. If poison gets in the eye, then you need to rinse out that area for 20 minutes.

If you were bit or stung by an insect or spider, then you need to get away from the nesting places of those insects and remove any stingers that are still in the skin. Clean the area out with soap and water and then apply an ice pack onto the area to reduce swelling. If bit on the arm or leg you should keep that area as close to the ground as possible to reduce the amount of venom that spreads.

Some species of snakes can be completely harmless where other species are extremely venomous. Snakes to look out for are the rattlesnake, cottonmouth, and copperhead. If bit by any snake check for symptoms of venom which include swelling, nausea, dizziness, fainting, weakness, convulsions, vomiting, diarrhea, rapid pulse, and loss of muscle coordination. If available, you should also add an antibiotic to the wound. It is also important if you can either take a picture of the snake or if you can safely kill it and bring it with you. This is so that if a medical team arrives you can show them what kind of snake it was and they will quickly know exactly which antivenom to use as all snakes have different types of venom. If no other option is available, you will want to quickly make a small incision above the area that was bitten and then suck on the wound in an effort to draw out the snake's venom.

In the United States, all poisonous snakes, save for the coral snake are what are known as pit vipers. As such, if you see a fat snake with a big head and slit pupils with what are known as heat pits on the end of their nose, then you know it is poisonous. As a general rule of thumb, if you come across a snake that is quite thin then you do not need to worry about it being poisonous. The coral snake is an exception to just about every rule regarding poisonous snakes, which means that you want to remember that if the pattern is red and black, it's safe Jack; meanwhile, if its red and yellow then it could kill you fellow.

Chapter 8: Food Preservation (Bonus Chapter)

In this bonus chapter from the first book in the Beginner to Badass series, "SHTF Prepping", we'll take a look at some of the best methods available for food preservation. This knowledge can be valuable for any aspiring adventurer that is planning on going out into the wild or to anyone that's interested in prepping food for unplanned disasters.

When it comes to canning, the goal is to keep an item in a state of maximum freshness for the greatest period of time possible. This can be accomplished either through what is known as water bath canning or via a process called pressure canning. If you have never canned anything before then you will likely want to start with water bath canning as it requires less specialized equipment while still giving you access to numerous different types of food to can, including tomatoes, jams, pickles, jellies and more. If you are planning on going whole hog and canning an entire meal, including meat, then pressure canning will be the better choice.

It doesn't matter which path you choose to head down, when you start canning you will always want to ensure the food you choose to can is as fresh and all-natural as possible. Likewise, you will want to ensure that it is free of blemish or bruising as this will shorten the shelf-life of the end result, defeating the purpose in the process. The best-case scenario is to choose items that have been prepared within the previous 12 hours, though if you have just picked a piece of fruit or vegetable off of the vine then you will want to let it ripen at least 24 hours before canning.

Above all else, however, it is important to be extremely careful when it comes to performing the canning process as, when done incorrectly, canning can lead to severe poisoning or even death. These hazardous issues are much more likely to occur when an unapproved method of canning is attempted, specifically via steam canning, oven canning or microwave canning as these processes do not allow the jars to reach the temperature required for true canning to occur. Always be based on a recipe and if your results show any visible irregularities dispose of them at once.

Prepare food for canning: Before you will be able to can your goods for maximum freshness, you are going to need to be to able pack them into jars properly. The first type of packing is what is known as raw packing and it is done by simply placing the items to be canned into the jars moments before the jars are going to be sealed. This process is most appropriate for vegetables that are going to be canned using a pressurized system. The other type of packing is what is known as hot packing and it is useful for a wider variety of foods than raw packing. This method of packing is done by simmering food in boiling water prior to placing it into jars. While it might not seem like much, it actually reduces the amount of air found in food, increasing its shelf life significantly. As an added bonus, the extra heat makes the seal the jar lid creates extra tight.

Water bath canning

Required tools

- Ladle

- Spatula

- Tongs

- An implement for removing jar lids from boiling water

- Two large pots

- One funnel

When it comes to performing this type of canning process, it is important to never move forward without having a recipe handy to refer to if you need additional guidance. You will want to start by placing both pots of water onto the stove over a pair of burners set to a high/medium heat. Add the jars as well as the lids to the water and let them boil for a minimum of ten minutes. After the ten minute mark, you will want to remove the jar from the pot and fill it as per the recipe's instructions, taking special care to keep all air bubbles out of the jar.

Once you have finished filling the jar, ensure that the mouth is clean before placing the lid on the jar, followed by the ring and ensure the seal is as strong as possible. Once the lid is on tight, the next step is to return it to the first pot and place it in water that is a minimum of 212 degrees F for the amount of time as indicated in the recipe. Finally, you will want to ensure the vacuum seal on each jar has been achieved prior to storing.

Tips for success

- Never place more than 6 cups of fruit into a jar for preserves as more than this amount will prevent the fruit from setting properly.

- If you are unsure about the quality of your water, use 2 T white vinegar to sterilize it. Avoid vinegar that has an acidity of greater than 5 percent.

- To prevent illness, you should avoid moving your jars for 24 hours after you have finished the canning process. Additionally, at the end of that period, if the lids have not popped to signify a strong seal then you know that something is wrong. Never use a lid more than once.

- The amount of time that you will need in order to process your jars will vary based on the altitude where the process takes place. If you are at between 1,000 and 3,000 feet, then you can expect the process to take about 5 minutes longer than it otherwise might. If you are above 3,000 feet but below 6,000 feet, then you can expect the process to take an extra 10 minutes and if you are above 6,000 feet then you can expect the process to take an extra 15 minutes.

Pressure canning

While you will use many of the same tools and techniques with pressure canning as you would with water bath canning, the pressure canner itself ends up making all of the difference. While there are countless different pressure canners available on the market today, you will want to ensure that the one you choose is large enough to hold at least 4 single quart jars as anything smaller than that will likely not be powerful enough to handle the tasks that you will want it to tackle.

Instructions: First and foremost, you are going to want to fill the canner full enough to ensure that while going through the process you do not run out of water. You will not need the jars to be completely submerged in this process. They cannot be totally dry either. Additionally, don't worry about sterilizing the lids or the jars, clean jars and lids will work just fine. They will need to be hot for the best results, however, this can be accomplished by placing a few inches of boiling water into each after they have been cleaned.

With the jars prepared, you are going to want to fill them as per the instructions in the recipe before adding them to the rack inside the pressure cooker. With the jars secured, you are going to want to replace the cover on the pressure cooker and heat it to the point that it boils. Once it starts boiling you will want to vent the steam for the first 10 minutes before closing the vent and letting the internal pressure build to the desired level. The amount of time you will want to leave the jars in the pressurized state will vary based on the recipe you are using. After the desired period of time has elapsed you will want to let the pressure canner cool for 12 hours prior to removing the jars.

As with water bath canning, the amount of pressure that you will need to use will vary based on your altitude. With a pressure canner, however, you will need to also consider if you are using a canner that is a weight gauge or one that is a dial gauge. If you are using a pressure canner with a dial gauge, and you are canning at 2,000 feet or below, then you will want to set your dial at 11. If you are above 2,000 feet and below 4,000 feet, then you will want to set your dial at 12. If you are above 4,000 feet and below 6,000 feet, then you will want to set your dial at 13. If you are above 6,000 feet and below 8,000 feet, then you will want to set your dial at 14. If, on the other hand, you are using a pressure canner with a weighted gauge then you will want to use the 10 setting if you are under 1,000 feet and the 15 setting if you are above 1,000 feet.

Fruit canning

When it comes to canning fruit, you can easily create your own canning syrup by combining sugar with water in a saucepan, adding a little heat and mixing well. If you want a light syrup, use two cups of sugar and one quart of water and if you want a thicker syrup use three cups sugar instead.

Apples: When it comes to canning apples, Granny Smith, Gala and Jona-Gold varieties tend to take to the process the most readily. Feel free to can apples using either canning method and keep in mind that 20 lbs. of apples will give you about 7.5 quarts canned. To properly prepare the apples, place them along with the syrup you have created into the second pot and let it boil. When it comes time to fill the jars, ensure that you leave about half an inch of space at the top of each, that each jar is free of air bubbles and that the mouth of each is clean. Finally, when it comes time to submerge the jars, do so for 20 minutes.

Cherries: It doesn't matter if you are canning sweet or sour cherries, the process is the same. It doesn't matter if they have pits or not, ten lbs. of cherries are likely to create four quarts of canned cherries. When it comes time to fill the jars, ensure that you leave about half an inch of space at the top of each, that each jar is free of air bubbles and that the mouth of each is clean. Finally, when it comes time to submerge the jars, do so for 25 minutes.

Peaches: You will find that roughly three pounds of peaches are needed to fill a quart jar. You will want to be sure that you boil the peaches for about 45 seconds, followed by an ice bath, prior to peeling to make the task much more manageable. Once they are peeled you will want to cover them in syrup immediately to prevent discoloration. Peaches remain just as delicious regardless if they are hot packed or raw packed, though if you choose to raw pack, be sure to fill as you go for the best results. On the other hand, if you are hot packing them you will want to cut the peaches directly into the syrup for the same results. When it comes time to fill the jars, ensure that you leave about half an inch of space at the top of each, that each jar is free of air bubbles and that the mouth of each is clean. Finally, when it comes time to submerge the jars, do so for 30 minutes.

Apricots: If you are planning to raw pack your apricots then you will not need to peel them, otherwise it is best that you do. Ten pounds of apricots will neatly fit into 9 pint jars. To prepare the apricots for the process you will want to slice them in half before placing them face down into the jars. When it comes time to fill the jars, ensure that you leave about half an inch of space at the top of each, that each jar is free of air bubbles and that the mouth of each is clean. Finally, when it comes time to submerge the jars, do so for 25 minutes.

Berries: It doesn't matter what types of berries that you favor, the canning process is always going to be the same.

You will always see better results when raw packing softer berries, though hard berries will be fine regardless. When it comes time to get down to it, you will find that 4 quart jars is enough for 15 lbs. of berries of all types. If you plan on hot packing your berries you will want to add in a quarter cup of sugar for each quart of berries before letting them sit for three hours prior to starting the process. When it comes time to fill the jars, ensure that you leave about half an inch of space at the top of each, that each jar is free of air bubbles and that the mouth of each is clean. Finally, when it comes time to submerge the jars, do so for 20 minutes.

Vegetable canning

Vegetables of all types require a pressure canner in order to be stored effectively, you will need to add 1 tsp. canning salt to each jar as well.

Tomatoes: You will find that roughly ten tomatoes fit in each quart jar and that it doesn't matter if you remove the skin or leave them natural prior to canning. When it comes time to fill the jars, ensure that you leave about half an inch of space at the top of each, that each jar is free of air bubbles and that the mouth of each is clean. Finally, when it comes time to submerge the jars, do so for 25 minutes.

Green beans: You will find that 10 lbs. of green beans fit neatly into eight quart jars and that raw packing and hot packing are equally successful. To prepare the beans you will want to break each in half and clean them thoroughly. If you plan on hot packing them you will want to allow the beans to boil for five minutes and then drain them before packing them into the jars loosely and then adding fresh boiling water. If you are raw packing the beans then you will want to pack as many as possible into each jar. When it comes time to fill the jars, ensure that you leave about an inch of space at the top of each, that each jar is free of air bubbles and that the mouth of each is clean. Finally, when it comes time to submerge the jars, do so for 25 minutes.

Corn: When you can corn, you will find that it takes approximately 30 lbs. to fit into seven quart jars and that corn takes longer to can than other vegetables. In order to can corn successfully you will want to blanch it and then add it to cool water for the best results. You will want to hot pack the corn for the best results; do so you will want to pack it into the jar loosely before adding the boiling water on top. Prior to hot packing, you will want to let the kernels simmer for about 5 minutes. When it comes time to fill the jars, ensure that you leave about an inch of space at the top of each, that each jar is free of air bubbles and that the mouth of each is clean. Finally, when it comes time to submerge the jars, do so for 90 minutes.

Carrots: You will always want to peel your carrots prior to canning to reduce your risk of botulism as much as possible. Two and a half pounds of carrots are required to fill a quart jar. If you plan on hot packing the carrots, you will want to simmer the carrots for about five minutes before packing them into the jars lightly and covering them in boiling water. When it comes time to fill the jars, ensure that you leave about an inch of space at the top of each, that each jar is free of air bubbles and that the mouth of each is clean. Finally, when it comes time to submerge the jars, do so for 30 minutes.

Potatoes: As with carrots, you will always want to peel your potatoes prior to canning to reduce your risk of botulism. Ten pounds of potatoes are required to fill seven quart jars. If you plan on hot packing the potatoes, you will want to simmer the potatoes for about five minutes before packing them into the jars lightly and covering them in boiling water. When it comes time to fill the jars, ensure that you leave about an inch of space at the top of each, that each jar is free of air bubbles and that the mouth of each is clean. Finally, when it comes time to submerge the jars, do so for 30 minutes.

Soup canning

Soup can only be canned effectively using the pressure canning method. When canning soup, you will want to avoid any additives such as noodles, milk, rice, flour or cream and to instead add those in after you have reheated the base. If you plan on including anything such as beans or peas, then you will want to cook them fully before canning them. When it comes to canning soup safely, ensure that all of the ingredients can be canned successfully individually for the best results.

Meat canning

When it comes to canning meat, you are going to want to keep a few things in mind for the best results. First and foremost, you will want to remove as much gristle and fat as possible while also ensuring the integrity of the cut of meat is top notch. You can either hot pack the meat in accompanying broth or raw pack it normally. It is important to never attempt to can meat via a water bath and only ever used canned meat that has been created using a pressure canner. The time required to pressure can meat is much longer than the times required for vegetables, but all of that time is needed to ensure things work out properly. Be patient and the results will be worth it.

Chapter 9: Water Preservation (Bonus Chapter)

In this second bonus chapter, you'll get to know about the best methods for preserving, storing, and finding water for long term survival after any natural or man-made disaster. While storing food will certainly come in handy, it will all be for naught if you don't have enough water to keep everyone you care about alive long enough to enjoy it. Luckily, there are plenty of different options when it comes to storing water in the long term, many of which are outlined below.

Find the right container: First things first, you are going to want to choose the right type of container to use for your water storage needs as not all containers, even those that hold water perfectly well in the short term, are fit for doing the job in the long term. While not all plastics should be used for long term water storage, those with the label of 2, 1, 4 and 5 all can be reliably used to store water for a prolonged period of time.

If you are thinking about storing your water in a glass container, then you are going to want to reconsider for a number of reasons. First and foremost, it can break easily and is even subject to microscopic flaws which can then hold bacteria, even if the container is cleaned on a regular basis. The only type of glass that can be used reliably is Pyrex, and even then, it is best to seek out alternatives instead whenever possible. All told, if you are looking to store a large amount of liquid for a prolonged period of time then stainless steel is going to be your best bet every single time. Stainless steel water containers are relatively common which means they can often be purchased quite cheaply and the water that stays within them can be considered safe for 40 years or more.

When it comes to storing your water safely in the long term it is important that you choose the right type of space for the best results. You are going to want to place it in a location that is structurally sound and unlikely to be in the path of the oncoming dangers you are hoping to prepare against. It should be someplace that is dry, cool and dark and the seal should remain unbroken until it is time to use the water to prevent contamination. Even then, if you have regular access to clean water then you will want to ensure that you swap out your reserves every six months to guarantee that things stay as clean and healthy as possible for when you really need it.

Clean your water: If you are storing a large amount of water for a prolonged period of time, then you are likely going to need to consider ways of keeping it clean if you need to replenish the source under less than ideal circumstances. The first thing you will always want to include is chlorine. If you are drawing water from the tap, then it will already have enough chlorine in it to sanitize it completely; if that is not the case then you will want to add in two drops of chlorine for every two liters of water that you are storing. When it comes time to choose the right bleach for the job, it is crucial that you choose one that is no more than 5 percent chlorine. Once you chlorinate your water you are going to want to ensure that the container remains open for at least an hour prior to consumption.

If you are dealing with larger amounts of water, a good choice to consider is instead what is known commonly as pool shock. More officially known as calcium hypochlorite, a single pound of this additive will clean up to ten thousand gallons of water without issue. When you are purchasing calcium hypochlorite you will need to ensure that it is less than 78 percent pure, while still being more than 68 percent pure. Additionally, you will need to ensure that it is free of water softeners.

If you find yourself in a scenario where you are unsure as to the quality of the water that is available for you to drink, then a good choice is to consider using iodine in it before drinking. If you are unsure about water that otherwise appears to be clear, then you will only need to use 5 drops per gallon. If, however, the water is murky in addition to being suspect, then you will need to use at least 10 drops per gallon to achieve the desired results.

Preparing for the long term

While an ample supply of water will get you through a short to moderate period without access to new clean water sources, eventually those supplies are going to run dry. If you find yourself in a scenario where this is a very real possibility, then you may need to consider the options outlined below if you do not have ready access to a well on any existing property.

Water filter: If you have ready access to water, just none of it readily drinkable, then looking into a water filter is a reasonable choice. Water filters come in all shapes and sizes, which means that there is bound to be one that is perfect for your needs on the market somewhere no matter how big, or small, they are. You can also find purifiers that purify for various levels of impurities including things like bacteria, salt, even radiation using either fiber filters, other types of small filters or a type of ceramic. There are even UV filters that work with a connected solar panel to ensure you always have access to powered water filtration. If you are worried that you won't be able to drink existing water, there is a type of water filter to allay your fears. When considering various types of water filters you will want to ensure that the one you choose doesn't require replaceable filters as that rather defeats the purpose.

Emergency still: If you are in a location that has access to lots of non-potable water then what is known as an emergency still is a practical choice. This type of device works by collecting water before boiling it to remove all impurities and then collecting the resulting steam so that it eventually turns back into water that has been highly purified. These types of devices are often much larger and more complicated than a simple filter but they leave the water drinkable indefinitely and can be used to withdraw water from damp soil, urine, even plant matter. If you find yourself in need of a variation of this device in a hurry, a sheet made of a thick plastic strung over the grouping of liquid and a hot day will provide much the same type of effect.

Water pump: If you are going to need to eventually draw water from an underground source then that means that you are going to need a water pump of some type. The most common water pumps are hand-operated and can then be rigged to run on everything from wind to animal power. If you are planning on using a hand pump, then you will need to determine just how deep you will have to go before you hit water. If your water table is below 40 feet, then you will need a deep pump instead of one that is rated as shallow.

Digging a well

If you don't have a well, but you do have a decent sized piece of property then there is a good chance that you have the capacity to create a well of your very own in many parts of the world. Digging your own well is not quick or easy but it can be extremely rewarding if you take the time to do it properly. Consider the following before you get started to ensure that your journey to dig a well isn't over before it even begins.

Know the area: While this might seem obvious, it is surprising how little many land owners know about their property. First and foremost, you need to be aware of any leach field or septic tanks that can be found on the property as bacteria from these types of areas can be found as much as 100 feet underground. Additionally, you will want to avoid all types of rocky outcroppings as they are generally a good indicator of additional rock underground that can make the process of digging infinitely more difficult and can cause the resulting water to have a strong mineral taste as well.

With the major hazards out of the way, you will then need to look into the details of the area and find out where the best place to begin actually is. If you're in the United States, the best place to start when it comes to finding details in your particular area is the US Geological Survey which can be accessed at Water.USGS.gov. With the specifics, out of the way, the next thing you will need to determine is what the local laws are like regarding the permits you will need to dig your own well if you are interested in keeping everything above board.

Digging a well: A hand dug well can be as simple or as complicated as you choose to make it. However, there are a few things that you will always want to keep in mind if you hope to have the easiest time of it possible. First and foremost, this means that you will want to line the top of your well also known as casing; this simply means surrounding the outer edge of the well with stones to prevent excessive contamination of the well. As an added bonus this will keep the opening of the well stable and help save your hard work from a cave-in. You will know that you are finished digging your hand dug well as soon as the bottom of your hole starts to fill with water.

Conclusion

Thank for making it through to the end of *Survival Skills: From Beginner to Badass. A Survival Guide with Life Saving Skills for the Wilderness or Any Dangerous Situation*, let's hope it was informative and able to provide you with all of the tools you need to achieve your survival goals, whatever it is that they may turn out to be. Just because you've finished this book doesn't mean there is nothing left to learn on the topic, as expanding your horizons is the only way to find the mastery you seek and there is always more information critical to your long-term survival that can be gleaned from somewhere, such as the other books in this series.

Remember, the most important thing that you can do in a survival situation is to remain calm and immediately asses your condition as well as your surroundings in an effort to determine just which of your primary needs you are going to need to take care of first. Many environments can be deceptively deadly and keeping on your guard at all times is always going to remain key, you never know when being on high alert might save your life. One of humanity's great strengths is its ability to adapt to virtually any situation; it's what has made us the dominant species on this planet and it is what can help you survive in any climate, in any situation. Always remember that survival should be viewed as a marathon instead of a sprint, and that slow and steady wins the race.

Survival is about more than just knowing the theory behind the scenario in question, it is about experiencing it in practice as well. All the books in the world won't help you when you find yourself in a real survival situation if you have never so much as pitched a tent in real life. Balance out your studies with real life experiences for the best results.

Finally, if you found this book useful in anyway, a review on Amazon is always appreciated!

www.ingramcontent.com/pod-product-compliance
Lightning Source LLC
Chambersburg PA
CBHW060159290526
45789CB00003B/1089